APPLE CIDER VINEGAR

The Natural Miracle Truth for Weight loss, Rejuvenate Hair, Skin, Body and Heart health.

By

Megan Lovefield

Table of Contents

WEIGHT LOSS AND APPLE CIDER VINEGAR	3
APPLE CIDER VINEGAR HAIRCARE BENEFITS	19
APPLE CIDER VINEGAR BEAUTY CARE BENEFITS	24
DIABETES AND APPLE CIDER VINEGAR	28
TUMMY ISSUES AND APPLE CIDER VINEGAR	32
HEART HEALTH AND APPLE CIDER VINEGAR	37
APPLE CIDER VINEGAR FOR ARTHRITIS	42

Weight loss and Apple cider vinegar

What is Apple Cider Vinegar?
Apple vinegar may be a popularly used as a primary ingredient in many natural remedies
for varied diseases. it's same that the legendary Greek medical man medical practitioner used it as associate all-in-one remedy for treating an inventory of diseases. Today, its known uses are for detoxification, treating respiratory disorder, and weight loss.

New medical analysis additionally suggests that apple vinegar intake will facilitate acid reflux, lower pressure level, improve polygenic disease and support weight loss. the advantages of apple vinegar come back from it's powerful healing compounds, that embody carboxylic acid, potassium, magnesium, probiotics and enzymes.

What's the MOTHER in Apple Cider Vinegar?

Apple vinegar with the mother is just unrefined, unpasteurized and unfiltered ACV. The "mother" could be a colony of useful microorganism, kind of like a Kombucha SCOBY, that helps produce vinegar through a secondary fermentation method. The mother" could be an advanced structure of useful acids that appear to own health advantages.

How to Use Apple Cider Vinegar for Weight Loss?

Apple cider vinegar has antioxidants and antibacterial properties that help in reducing cellular inflammation and infections. It is just superb for promoting overall health.

You could also be interested in trying out the ACV diet for shedding belly fat and improving overall health.

The easiest way to use ACV for shedding weight is to have 1 tablespoon raw organic apple cider vinegar mixed in a cup of water and drink it on an empty stomach in the morning. Ideally, you should be having 2 tablespoons of vinegar to a cup of water and have it 1 -3 times a day. But it is not easy for all to drink it that way for its funny taste. The maximum weight loss results with ACV can be achieved when it is combined with other fat burning diets or as part of other recipes.

Apple Cider Vinegar weight loss drinks and recipes.

1. ACV and Maple Syrup Mixture
Unrefined syrup contains antioxidants, helpful nutrients, and phytochemicals than the ketohexose syrup or white sugar. Adding syrup in ACV makes the drink palatable and sweet while not adding dangerous calories to that. Taka a glass of warm water and add to it 1 tablespoon apple cider vinegar and sweeten the drink with 1 tablespoon maple syrup. Instead of plain water, you can use green tea with ACV and maple syrup for better fat burning results.

2. ACV and Water
Drinking two cups of water mixed with ACV before meals is nice for appetency suppression and up metabolism.

Usage Direction: Take two cups (5ooml) of water and add one tablespoon ACV in it; drink this ACV mixed water half-hour before the meal. it's the only apple vinegar weight loss drink.

3. Apple Cider Vinegar and Honey

Honey and ACV is that the ancient health "elixir" suggested by Hippocrates of Greece. you'll conjointly mix the health 'elixir' with alternative flavor ingredients illustrious for his or her fat burning quality. Here are unit some the most effective combinations:

a) Combine 2 tablespoons of honey in Associate in Nursing equal quantity of ACV and add this mixture to eight Oz of water and drink it. Honey not solely sweetens the drink however conjointly brings several health edges with it. it's best to possess this drink half-hour before the meal.

b) Use vinegar and honey combine as a dressing or mix it into fruit juices

c) Take a glass of water and increase it one tablespoon apple cider vinegar, two teaspoon Honey, a pinch of cayenne pepper, ½ teaspoon garlic paste, and five drops of lemon juice; stir the mixture well and drink half-hour before the meal. This drink is nice suppressing appetency and up metabolism and fat burning.

d) Add two teaspoon Honey and one teaspoon ACV in one cup of freshly brewed green tea and drink it three times daily. tea will suppress appetency and increase the speed of metabolism.

4. ACV and Cinnamon

Cinnamon contains glorious natural ingredients that facilitate to balance the blood glucose. the mixture of ACV, cinnamon powder, honey and juice is effective for weight loss and overall improvement of health. Usage Direction: Take a cup of water and increase it 2 tablespoons organic apple vinegar, one tablespoon honey, ½ teaspoon cinnamon powder and few drops recent juice. Stir the juice well and drink it half-hour before the meal daily.

5. Apple Cider Vinegar Dressed Salad

Make a dish with a pair of tomatoes, a pair of cut cucumbers and three sliced onions. Dress the dish with a mix of two Oz every ACV and water, a pair of teaspoon sugar, ¼ teaspoon black pepper and salt as required. ingestion ACV dressed dish often with the meal can facilitate in shedding weight quickly.

6. Additional Ways to Use ACV for Weight Loss

Here are a couple of easy apple vinegar weight loss recipes and diets:

- Use ACV with olive oil for salad dressing; it tastes great especially the leafy green salads
- Mix 2 tablespoons of ACV with orange juice
- Use with flaxseed and honey to create a power salad dressing.
- Use ACV for pickling vegetables and raw fruits
- Substitute ordinary cooking vinegar with ACV
- Use a little ACV when you are making any fermented food items.

Tips and Warnings on ACV Diet

- If you utilize the ACV justly, you'll be able to expect to induce sensible weight loss results with it however the incorrect usage can cause side effects at constant time. Here are some tips and warnings for ACV use:
- Limit the daily intake of apple cider vinegar to 2 or 3 tablespoons per day; start off with 1

teaspoon per day and then gradually increase the intake as your body gets accustomed to tolerating ACV
- Always dilute the ACV in water, drink, or honey
- Take the apple cider vinegar weight loss drinks 30 minutes before the meal
- Use only the raw, organic, unpasteurized and unfiltered ACV
- The effectiveness of ACV for weight loss do not have any scientific backing
- Overdose of ACV can cause hypokalemia which leads to osteoporosis (poor born density)
- ACV is not recommended for patients using laxatives, prescription medicines or diuretics
- Do not use undiluted ACV as it may damage tooth enamel and cause burn to the esophagus, dyspepsia, nausea, and pyrosis
- Follow a balanced diet and do physical exercises to achieve maximum weight loss results with ACV diet
- Some might experience an allergic reaction such as itching, swelling, rash, respiratory issues, etc.

when ACV intake; discontinue this diet in such cases.
- Certainly, apple cider vinegar is a wise choice to make because of the many health benefits you achieve from this natural diet. It detoxifies the body and improves the antimicrobial immunity of the body. Regular intake of ACV proved to be beneficial for preventing diabetes, cardiovascular diseases, cancer, bad cholesterol, inflammation, acid reflux, indigestion and many other common illnesses.
- You if you have not tried it, start taking apple cider vinegar weight loss drinks and recipes

The weight loss benefit from apple cider vinegar (ACV).

Unlike the various craze diets and supplements for fast fat loss that comes and goes, the ACV is a tested natural supplement that may assist you to melt off step by step and steady.

The vinegar obtained from doubly hard apples additionally has many preventative and curative health advantages.

In this article, we tend to shall have a detailed explore the 'apple vinegar weight loss diets' effectiveness and also the right thanks to use this vinegar for shedding pounds naturally.

1.Apple Cider Vinegar Is a Good Appetite Suppressor

The analysis report revealed within the European Journal of Clinical Nutrition in 2005 indicates the effectiveness of apple vinegar diet in craving suppression.

According to the on top of study, the participants UN agency had bread and apple vinegar were less hungry compared to others UN agency had solely the bread. The carboxylic acid gift in ACV makes the person feel fuller and suppresses the craving for several hours.

There is additionally proof that indicate that persons UN agency consume a tablespoon of ACV half-hour before the meals have lowered craving for food and eat less throughout meals

The cellulose substance gift in apples and ACV reduces the craving and makes an individual feel fuller with a lesser quantity of food intake. AN apple contains concerning one.5 grams of cellulose substance.

2.Helps in Maintaining Blood Sugar Balance

The blood glucose level contains a heap to try and do with our appetence and consumption habits that acts as a determinative in avoirdupois.

Sudden spike and crashes in blood glucose level produce the urge in United States to nibble at food between meals. only if the blood glucose level is stable, we will follow the healthy diet and consumption habits.

Study reports on ACV indicated that persons who took the vinegar had lower glucose level once the meals.

Studies additionally showed that one that took higher quantity of ACV were ready to maintain a balanced level of glucose even ninety minutes once the meal.

3.ACV Diet Increases the Rate of Metabolism

Improved metabolism leads to faster fat burning that is essential for weight loss.

The organic acids and enzymes contained within the apple vinegar are sensible for promoting higher levels of healthy metabolism.

One of the studies conducted in 2009 in Japan within which ethanoic acid was given to rats that were consumed a diet with high fats. The results of the study showed that lesser fat accumulation in rats that were fed with ethanoic acid.

Even though there are not many studies on this yet, it is assumed that people who consume ACV rich in acetic acid would experience improved metabolic rate and faster fat burning.

4. Promotes Healthy Insulin Functioning

It is the correct quantity of hypoglycemic agent endocrine production and also the offer of it into the blood streams that ensures the immediate conversion of blood glucose into energy required by the body. Healthy functioning of hypoglycemic agent endocrine not solely reduces the fat storage within the body however additionally reduces the probabilities of sort two polygenic disorder.

The apple vinegar diet helps improved production and functioning of hypoglycemic agent endocrine. The organic acids within the apple vinegar have an understandable impact keep the blood glucose levels in balance; this additionally helps in minimizing the dangerous effects of sort two diabetics.

Apple vinegar for weight loss works well by enhancing the hypoglycemic agent potency and regulation within the body.

5. ACV Is Good for Detoxifying the Body

One of the most reasons for poor metabolism is that the presence of high quantity of poison within the body.

It is found that that regular consumption of apple vinegar helps in flushing out the toxins from the body, particularly those accumulated within the colon. This vinegar conjointly detoxifies the liver.

If reality most of the body detoxifying, drinks and tonics contain apple vinegar because the one amongst the main ingredients in them.

Results of Apple Cider Vinegar diet for Weight Loss

There are unit variety of studies that indicate the effectiveness of apple vinegar for weight loss.

The enzymes and organic acids gift within the ACV has nice influence on promoting healthy metabolism that reduces the fat storage within the fat cells of the body.

As we've got mentioned higher than, it helps US to eat less because it suppresses the craving. ACV additionally reduces the surplus water retention within the body; it results in shedding of weight because of high water retention.

Vinegar has properties that facilitate to stay the glucose at moderate levels even when the meals. A teaspoon or 2 of ACV consumption before the meals is nice because it would facilitate in reduced usage of hypoglycemic agent secretion for glucose metabolism.

It is true that the load loss result from the ACV is proscribed, however the regular consumption of it'll maintain steady reduction of weight.

Going the by the final observation on the results given by numerous studies on ACV for weight loss, daily 2 spoons vinegar consumption can cause fifteen to twenty pounds weight loss in one year amount. You cannot expect speedy weight loss results with apple vinegar diet; the fat loss results are gradual and steady over a period.

How to use Apple Cider Vinegar for Weight Loss?

Most people could notice it arduous to consume the ACV in undiluted type for its harsh style and acidity. Most of the house remedies suggest diluting one or 2 teaspoons of ACV into a glass of water and drink it before every meal.

For some individuals, it should take an extended time to urge accustomed ACV diet.

As you start to use apple acetum diet for weight loss, you'll be able to begin with a teaspoon quantity of it for every week and so step by step increase the intake up to a pair of tablespoons daily in a month's time

The best weight loss result's attainable once ACV is consumed regarding 3o minutes before the meals. Some natural remedy practitioners suggest a tablespoon of ACV intake in empty stomachs within the morning for optimum advantages.

People with high acidity problems could notice it tough to follow this diet; in such cases, it's smart to require the opinion of a doctor before beginning this diet.

It is smart to avoid the intake of undiluted vinegar because the robust organic acids in it should harm teeth and irritate/hurt the tender tissues in throat and muscle system.

Tips on Getting Best Results from Apple Cider Vinegar Weight Loss Diet

- Like any alternative weight loss diet, you cannot expect smart fat loss results with apple vinegar diet while not healthy diets and physical workouts at the side of it.
- It is necessary that you just maintain low calories and diet.
- Let your diet contain additional of macromolecule, whole grains, vegetables, and fruits as they will offer your body healthy quantity of vitamins and nutrients needed for the body while not too several calories and fat.
- Strictly avoid all refined and processed food for higher weight loss results from ACV diet. it's conjointly necessary to avoid soda and soft drinks as they are rich in calories.
- Make sure to drink a minimum of eight glasses of water daily because it won't solely suppress the appetency however conjointly necessary for healthy metabolism and association of the body.

- Regular physical exercises (intense cardio exercises) are vital for burning further calories deposits within the body.
- If you are doing not have the time and convenience to have interaction in workouts at a gymnasium, at least, take three miles of brisk walking or cardiopulmonary exercise for 3 to 5 times every week.
- You can lose, at least, ten pounds a month with 'apple drink weight loss diet if you'll follow up with correct diet and exercise.

Apple cider vinegar haircare benefits

Apple Cider Vinegar does deliver when it comes to hair care. For those dealing with hair issues such as itchy scalp or hair breakage, apple cider vinegar might be a great natural remedy to explore.

Why use ACV for hair care?

Acidity and pH scale
For one, apple vinegar on the far side having some well-researched health properties is associate acidic substance. It contains sensible amounts of carboxylic acid.

Hair that appears uninteresting, brittle, or kinky tends to be a lot of alkalescent or higher on the ph. The concept is that associate acid substance, like ACV, helps lower pH scale and brings hair health into balance.

Antimicrobial

ACV is additionally a well-liked home disinfectant. it's going to facilitate management the bacterium or fungi that may result in scalp and hair issues, admire minor infections or itch.

Other claims

Apple vinegar is praised for being made in vitamins and minerals sensible for hair, like antioxidant and B. Some conjointly claim it contains alpha-hydroxy acid that helps exfoliate scalp skin, which it's medication, which might facilitate with dandruff.

Benefits of Apple Cider Vinegar for your Hair

1. Balances the hair's pH scale. bound hair product disrupt the hair's pH scale. ACV will bring the hair's pH scale back to best levels as a result of it naturally has constant pH scale as healthy hair.

2. Rejuvenates the hair with its cleansing and elucidative properties. ACV removes clumpy residue from hair product build up.

3. Adds shine to the hair. ACV closes the hair cuticle, that helps it to mirror lightweight and makes hair shiny.

4. Reduces crimp/ frizz. Again, once the scales of the hair don't lay flat, the hair begins to dry out and become curly.
Reduces restless scalp and dandruff (especially as a result of dry, winter air).
5. Prevents split ends. That's why it's nice to treat your hair with ACV once you're obtaining on the brink of your next haircut and area unit starting to have split ends.
6. Detangles the hair. because it smooths out the cuticles, it detangles the hair and might be an honest different to hair conditioner.
7. Encourages hair growth. It treats clogged hair follicles and stimulates higher circulation on the pinnacle which can stimulate hair growth or stop hair loss.
8. Packed with nutrients. ACV contains nutrients useful to the hair as well as B vitamins, vitamin C, and K.
9. It's medication which might forestall scalp-related conditions like dandruff or different conditions that cause dry flaky scalp.

Apple Cider Vinegar Rinse Recipe

This simple ACV rinse recipe can be used one to two times weekly. While some say you can use it as a conditioner, I use it in addition to conditioner because my hair gets tangled. If you have dry hair you may want to use a little less ACV and if you have oily hair, then you may want to use a bit more.

Ingredients

2 Tbsp. raw organic apple cider vinegar
1 cup water

Directions

1. Combine ingredients in a cup or bowl.
Shampoo and condition as you normally would. Once you've rinsed both the shampoo and conditioner, cover your hair with the raw apple cider vinegar rinse. (Be sure to close your eyes tightly.)
Rinse your hair thoroughly.

Tips:

Don't be so concerned about the smell of ACV because once it dries, your hair will no longer smell like vinegar.

You may also want to try using a squeeze bottle to more evenly apply ACV, rather than a bowl or cup which provides less even application. (I used a bowl but may use a squeeze next time.)

You can experiment with using the ACV instead of hair conditioner, rather than in addition to it. You may not need both.

Apple cider vinegar beauty care benefits

Skin Toner
Psoriasis sufferers praise apple cider vinegar for reducing inflammation. Apply a few drops to a cotton ball and rub on your T-zone or other dry spots to prevent breakouts and minimize blemishes.

Reduce Age Spots
Apple Cider Vinegar contains sulfur that fights the effects of aging, including age spots. Dab age spots, or liver spots, with ACV every night before you go to sleep. Do not wash off the vinegar. If you feel a stinging sensation, dilute the vinegar with water. Wash off in the morning.

Acne Remedy
ACV kills bacteria and balances skin's pH level. It also absorbs excessive oil from our skin, which is a leading cause of acne. Mix one part vinegar to 3-4 parts water.

Apply solution directly to your skin with clean cotton pad, and leave it there for about ten minutes. After ten minutes, rinse off the vinegar. Repeat this three times a day. For severe cases of acne, the solution can be used overnight without rinsing.

Teeth Whitener

Gargle with apple cider vinegar in the morning. The vinegar helps remove stains, whiten teeth, and kill bacteria in your mouth and gums. Brush as usual after you gargle.

Sunburn Relief

Relieve the pain of a sunburn and minimize peeling by applying a wash cloth soaked in apple cider vinegar to the area.

Vein Pain

ACV is great for varicose veins because it improves circulation in the vein wall and helps to ease the bulging and swelling vein so it is less noticeable and less painful. Combine equal parts ACV and your favorite lotion. Apply morning and night to varicose veins in a circular motion until absorbed. Depending on the severity of your varicose veins, you should begin to see improvement within a month.

Natural Deodorant

Most commercial deodorants are antiperspirants, which block your ability to sweat. Since sweat is one of your body's natural means of detoxification, blocking your ability to sweat can block your ability to detoxify. ACV absorbs and neutralizes odors. Simply rub a bit of ACV in your underarms. The vinegary smell dissipates once it dries.

Wart Removal

Try placing a cotton pad soaked in apple cider vinegar on top, then secure with a bandage. Leave on overnight and remove in the morning. If you stick to this consistently for a week, you should start to see results.

Soothing Bath Soak

The next time you get ready to slip into a warm bath, add one to two capfuls of apple cider vinegar. It draws toxins out of the body, leaving behind toned and moisturized skin.

Foot and Skin Fungus

Just as ACV can help kill Candida in the body, it is often useful against yeast and fungus on the skin and nails. If you have foot or toe fungus, soak the feet in 1 cup of ACV in water or apply directly to the affected area. For skin fungus or yeast, apply ACV directly. For children or those with sensitive skin, it is best to dilute the ACV with water before applying to the skin.

Eliminates Bad Breath

Add a 1/2 tablespoon of ACV to a cup of water. Then, gargle for 10 seconds at a time until the cup is completely empty.

Invigorating Foot Soak

Use apple cider vinegar to soothe aching and swollen feet.

Facial Mask

Mix equal parts apple cider vinegar and bentonite clay, add 1 tablespoon raw honey. Apply to skin. Leave this detoxifying, deep-pore treatment on for 10-15 minutes before rinsing off with warm water.

Diabetes and Apple cider vinegar

Type two Diabetes may be a preventable and chronic disease that affects however your body controls sugar (glucose) in your blood. Medications, diet, and exercise are the quality treatments. however recent studies vouch for one thing you'll be able to realize in most room cupboards too: That is apple cider vinegar.

Apple cider vinegar has been used for centuries and is made from fermented apple mash. It contains acetic acid, vitamins, minerals, amino acids, polyphenols and other types of acids. The "mother" fluid is a product of a long fermentation process and will often look cloudy because of the non-infectious and non-toxic bacteria (the probiotics) that it contains. Other, "non-mother" products are filtered to remove the cloudiness and may be less beneficial. Evidence is beginning to pile up for at least some uses of apple cider vinegar commonly known as ACV. Many professionals will recommend, however, that you only use the "mother" ACV and not any filtered ACV products.

ACV and fasting blood sugar levels

ACV may even be beneficial for helping to regulate fasting blood sugar levels which are your blood sugar levels after a period of fasting. These levels are most often determined when you wake up in the morning before you eat anything.

In a study published in *Diabetes Care*, researchers studied the effects of two tablespoons of ACV at bedtime to determine if ACV had an effect on fasting blood glucose.

The results of the study showed that two tablespoons of ACV at bedtime helped to regulate fasting blood glucose levels in patients with type II diabetes.

How Much ACV Should You Take for Diabetes?

• Although the results of ACV vary from one individual to subsequent, if you concentrate on most of the studies regarding ACV, then a tablespoon or 2 looks to be sufficient to get the advantages related to ACV and glucose regulation.

• To facilitate regulate blood glucose once a meal, adding 2 tablespoons of ACV to your dressing or to a

glass of water might be sufficient to assist regulate blood glucose levels once your meal.
• For the aim of regulation fast blood glucose levels, 2 tablespoons of vinegar at bed time may even be useful for regulation your blood glucose levels whereas you sleep.
• Adding 2 tablespoons of ACV to a glass of water before time of day may so assist you to manage blood glucose levels.
• As a general note, don't consume undiluted ACV because it erodes solid body substance and may cause burns to the sensitive tissues within the mouth and throat.

Honey and ACV

Many people wish to add honey to their ACV to offset the acidic style and to relish the combined health edges of ACV and honey.

Although honey offers some health edges, it's necessary to grasp that honey is usually sugar and it will increase your calorie and saccharide intake. For managing polygenic disorder, honey ought to be calculated as a part of your total saccharide intake. Various studies on honey showed that it should not have identical impact on blood glucose levels as sugar will. If you've got well-managed polygenic disorder, don't seem to be overweight and square measure otherwise healthy, then honey as a replacement for sugar is useful.

If you've got any doubt, it's best to ask your doctor.

Tummy issues and Apple cider vinegar

Apple Cider Vinegar (ACV) is a more effective treatment for stomach pain than many of the old standbys, such as antacids. You've probably been told that stomach pain and related ailments are caused largely by excess acid and, in turn, need to be treated using an antacid.

Actually, this is just the opposite of how an acid stomach should be treated. The stomach is naturally acidic, so pain occurs because of an imbalance or lack of acid in the stomach.

Apple Cider Vinegar (ACV) is high in pectin content. Without getting too scientific on you, pectin is part of a plant's biology and it helps to form fibrous matter in your stomach. This aids in preventing diarrhea. Pectin also does a wonderful job of forming a protective coat around the colon_lining. This is quite soothing and is really helpful in those times you are suffering from intestinal spasms.

Why Should I Use Apple Cider Vinegar for Indigestion?

Apple cider vinegar is a safe, natural treatment that is very effective for relieving stomach cramping and pain. It also helps to alkalize bodily pH, assisting the body in fighting the underlying cause of the problem.

How to Take Apple Cider Vinegar for Stomach Pain?

To cure most stomach pain and nausea, drink 1-2 tablespoons of organic apple cider vinegar straight from the bottle.

If you experience regular stomach issues, try drinking a tonic of one teaspoon to two tablespoons of ACV in a large glass of water with each meal. You'll experience relief from stomach pain and gain better health all around.

How to Take Apple Cider Vinegar for Upset Stomach:

ACV is a natural bacteria combatant to settle an upset stomach. Read on to find out the various ways of using ACV along with other natural ingredients.

Apple Cider Vinegar and Water for Upset Stomach:

- ACV's alkaline effect alleviates various the stomach pain and discomfort. Reap in all the goodness of ACV with this simple mix of 2 tablespoons of ACV into a cup of warm water. This mixture can be consumed prior to having your food.
- Apple Cider Vinegar and Baking Soda for Upset Stomach:
- When stomach acids are neutralized, it helps proper digestion. This is what baking soda does. Baking soda along with ACV causes a carbonation effect and thus promotes burping, to relieve excess gas. To one cup of water, mix 1teaspoon of ACV and half a teaspoon of baking soda. Consume this solution immediately.

Apple Cider Vinegar and Honey for Upset Stomach:

Honey and ACV mix is very effective to soothe issues like stomach cramps, indigestion and heart burn. Make this concoction using a cup of water, and adding 1 table spoon each of ACV and honey. Stir it well and drink.

Apple Cider Vinegar Fruit Drink for Upset Stomach:

ACV being so versatile that it works very well with other natural ingredients. To help soothe the stomach cramps and pains associated with upset stomach, ACV can be mixed with any fruit juices. Hence prevent upset stomach by adding a teaspoon full of ACV to your favorite fruit juices and consume this before meals.

Apple Cider Vinegar and Tea for Upset Stomach:

Well known for its antioxidants and anti-inflammatory properties, green tea treats upset stomach and stomach aches. Combining this with ACV helps not only to evade the discomfort caused by upset stomach, but also promotes healthy digestion. For making this recipe, prepare your green tea as usual and dilute a teaspoon of ACV into it. Stir well and consume this mixture.

Apart from its healing properties, Apple Cider Vinegar is well known for its culinary usage. Incorporate ACV into your diet by using it as a salad dressing. Its sour taste adds tanginess and freshness to your salad. It is quite surprising and to hear about this key ingredient ACV and its benefits to heal many of health issues.

Heart health and Apple cider vinegar

Apple cider vinegar (ACV) is heart healthy and has a multitude of other health benefits. It really works for people who is having heart blockage and heart disease.

Who Can Use,
1) People diagnosed with Heart blockage, Heart Disease
2) People who cannot afford By - Pass Surgery or can't go for By - Pass Surgery.
3) Prevention of Repeated Heart Attacks
4) Suffering from Constipation, Ulcers
5) People who are looking for Weight loss

I recommend you try this super heart tonic to detox and cleanse your heart from blockage and heart disease.

THIS SUPER HEART TONIC IS MADE WITH GINGER, GARLIC, HONEY, LEMON JUICE & APPLE CIDER VINEGAR

Garlic Health Benefits:
Reduce Blood Pressure, Anti Block, Reduces Cholesterols, Anti-Bacterial Properties, Reduces Sugar Level, Treats Skin Infection, Reduce Weight, Treats Respiratory problems and many more.

Ginger Health Benefits:
Preventing and curing heart disease, increase blood flow, reduces weight, increase energy, Good for cold, cough and many more.

Lemon Health Benefits:
Regulates Heart Beat, Helps in Proper Functioning of Heart, Reduces Weight and many more.

Apple Cider Health Benefits:
Remove Toxins from body, contains minerals, potassium, vitamins and enzymes.

Honey Health Benefits:
Reduces Cholesterol, Fights Bacteria, Energize Body, Anti-Oxidants, Reduce Risk of Cancer & Heart Disease.

This drink is so easy to put together. You have to extract the juice from the ingredients. Mix all up, heat it up, cool it down and add honey. That's it.

How to Consume:
Drink 1 tablespoon of this tonic, Empty Stomach in Morning. You can also have 1 tablespoon in the afternoon and night.

How long can this be stored:
This can be stored in fridge for 1 to 2 months. Use clean dry spoons when handling.

Preparation Time: 30 mins
Cooking Time: 30 mins
Makes: 5 cups of Drink
Ingredients:

- Ginger Juice - 1 cup
- Garlic Puree - 1 cup
- Lemon Juice - 1 cup
- Apple Cider Vinegar - 1 cup
- Organic Honey - 3 cup

- **(YOU CAN USE ANY CUP, USE THE SAME CUP TO MEASURE ALL THE INGREDIENTS)**

Method:
1. Take ginger juice, garlic juice, lemon juice, vinegar in a sauce pan and cook on medium heat for 30 mins. Keep mixing.

2. Take it off heat, cool it completely.

3. Add in 3 cups of honey and mix well.

4. Pour this in a clean bottle and store in fridge.

Promotes Healthy Cholesterol
Not only does apple cider vinegar support healthy cholesterol, studies have shown that it can protect from arterial damage or oxidation, which is the main risk of high cholesterol.

Promotes Healthy Blood Sugar
Studies have shown that apple cider vinegar has strong anti-glycemic properties that support a healthy blood sugar level. The vinegar actually blocks some of the digestion of starch, preventing it from raising your blood sugar.

Has Antioxidant Properties
Apple cider vinegar contains many antioxidants to help keep your body healthy and running smoothly, including catechin, gallic acid, caffeic and chlorogenic acids.

Improves Nutrient Absorption
The acetic acid in apple cider vinegar can increase your body's absorption of important minerals from the food you eat. Adding vinegar to your salad dressing may also help you absorb more nutrients from your leafy greens!

Apple Cider Vinegar for Arthritis

Apple vinegar will reduce the pain and swelling of the joints that characterizes differing types of inflammatory disease. However, not all sorts of apple vinegar area unit effective. you wish to use pure vinegar naturally hard from apple potable. As a matter of truth, any potable or alternative carbohydrate-rich liquids which will be become alkyl radical alcohol (ethanol) by fermentation are often additional hard to induce vinegar. it always undergoes filtering and pasteurization before showing on search shelves. This process robs the vinegar of the many of its natural healing properties. Use raw, organic apple vinegar that's unfiltered and unprocessed. It ought to contain what's known as the "mother of vinegar," which provides the liquid a cloudy look. it's a full of life advanced of polysaccharides, acetic acid, microorganism and fungi that still turn out B-complex vitamins and alternative useful compounds. In fact, you'll use this to form vinegar from fruit crush or potable.

Which type of inflammatory disease are often treated with apple potable vinegar?
There are unit over 100 varieties and subtypes of inflammatory disease. In fact, inflammatory disease merely means that inflammation of joints; it often because of varied reasons. However, degenerative arthritis, atrophic arthritis, arthritis and rheumatoid arthritis area unit a number of the foremost usually seen joint issues.

Osteoarthritis

This age-associated chronic condition affects major joints corresponding to hips, knees, and hands. degenerative joint disease results from the mechanical wear and tear of the joint structures, significantly the gristle that covers the ideas of bones. principally poignant old and older individuals, it's a serious reason behind loss of movement and incapacity. Since this condition is irreversible, and therefore the solely definitive treatment may be a joint replacement, the main target is on managing the pain and discomfort and reducing more deterioration. That's wherever apple cider vinegar comes in.

How to use ACV for osteoarthritis:
• Taking the vinegar, beside some raw honey to form it additional appetizing, is one amongst the most effective home remedies for degenerative joint disease.
• Add 1-2 tablespoons of ACV to plain water or associate degree herb tea and sweeten the drink with honey in an exceedingly 1:1 or 2:1 quantitative relation looking on your tolerance. you would possibly see a major distinction in as very little as a number of weeks of victimization this remedy.

Rheumatoid inflammatory disease
This type of inflammatory disease is sort of common and is characterized by stiffness within the joints in the middle of pain and marked reduction in vary of motion of the affected joints. It will have an effect on anyone, regardless of age. The stiffness affects the little joints additional typically and is additional marked within the morning. Prolonged joint stiffness collectively gets out of bed is, in fact, the distinguishing feature of this diseases. This associate degree response condition can have an effect on internal organs similarly.

The exact cause of rheumatoid arthritis is not known, but free radical damage and toxins accumulating in the body are considered risk factors. Mineral deficiencies, especially the deficiency of calcium and magnesium exacerbate the condition. Conventional treatment involves taking certain drugs referred to as disease-modifying anti-rheumatic drugs or DMARDs as well as steroidal or non-steroidal anti-inflammatory drugs. These drugs help reduce the inflammation of the joints and pain, but they do have grave side effects, especially when used long-term.

Apple cider vinegar has been found to be very effective in relieving the painful symptoms of this condition. Being a good diuretic and laxative, apple cider vinegar helps eliminate toxins from the body. It is also rich in antioxidant substances that help counteract free radical damage that triggers immune reactions.
Apple cider vinegar contains minerals calcium, magnesium, potassium, iron and phosphorus and some vitamins. The mineral content in the vinegar may be low, but what's important is that it promotes the absorption of minerals from food. Vinegar

containing 'mother' is an excellent prebiotic that helps the intestinal flora. These microbes residing in the intestines are thought to play a serious role in immune modulation.

How to use ACV for rheumatoid arthritis:
- Besides drinking apple cider vinegar with honey once or twice a day, you can use it topically for local pain relief.
- Add 2 cups of ACV to your bath water and sit in it for 30 minutes before going to bed. This will help reduce morning stiffness.
- A mixture of the vinegar in oil can be used externally on affected joints to bring relief. Add two parts of apple cider vinegar to 1 part of coconut oil or olive oil and massage the mixture in.

Gout

Gout is a cause of the joint pain and inflammation of the joints, especially in the limbs, when uric acid crystals accumulate. Excess uric acid in the blood due to the breakdown of purines that come from certain protein-rich foods such as meat and seafood, and its inefficient removal by the kidneys, is the main cause of gout. It is a very painful condition, often appearing suddenly, sometimes in sleep. People who have gout often report that regular use of apple cider vinegar help avoid episodes.

The acetic acid content of the vinegar is thought to be the main agent here. It alkalizes the body and helps neutralize the uric acid and prevents the formation of needle-like crystals.

How to use ACV for gout:
- A classic gout-relief recipe is taking 2 tablespoon of apple cider vinegar in a cup of water twice a day. Make sure that the vinegar is natural, unfiltered, and unpasteurized, and that it contains the 'mother.'
- To get immediate pain relief at the site of inflammation, cover the area with a washcloth dipped in apple cider vinegar. Soaking your feet in a foot bath containing 1 cup vinegar in 4 cups warm water also helps.

Psoriatic arthritis

This is a type of arthritis most commonly seen in people who have active psoriasis or family history of this disorder. Psoriasis usually appears as patches of dry, flaky skin with itching or burning sensation. When occurring on the scalp, psoriasis often looks like an aggressive form of dandruff. Apple cider vinegar has a long history of being used topically to relieve the itching and burning, and it is reportedly quite effective.

People who have psoriatic arthritis often fail to get a correct diagnosis. The exact cause of psoriasis is not known, but it is considered an autoimmune condition like rheumatoid arthritis. Even if it's correctly diagnosed, there's no curative treatment for either psoriasis or psoriatic arthritis, so these conditions are often treated with immune-suppressing drugs. If one already has psoriasis and then develops pain in the joints, it is a good idea to use apple cider vinegar regularly.

How to use ACV for psoriatic arthritis:
- Apple cider vinegar can be incorporated into your daily diet by using it for pickling and as salad dressing in place of white vinegar. It offers many other health benefits like blood sugar control in diabetics and pre-diabetics and weight reduction. Since diabetes and obesity are known risk factors for arthritis, it may indirectly help reduce the symptoms. The effectiveness of apple cider vinegar can be further enhanced by mixing it with other naturally anti-inflammatory foods such as ginger, garlic, cinnamon, tart cherry juice and grape juice.

As you can see Apple Cider Vinegar Is Awesome and a Miracle wonder for your body! Use it in your daily routine for your health, beauty and hair routine, weight loss, heart health…extra!

www.ingramcontent.com/pod-product-compliance
Lightning Source LLC
Chambersburg PA
CBHW080111100225
21681CB00015B/1596